Pescatarian Cooking Guide

Quick and straightforward Healthy Delicious Dishes for your everyday meals

Lara Dillard

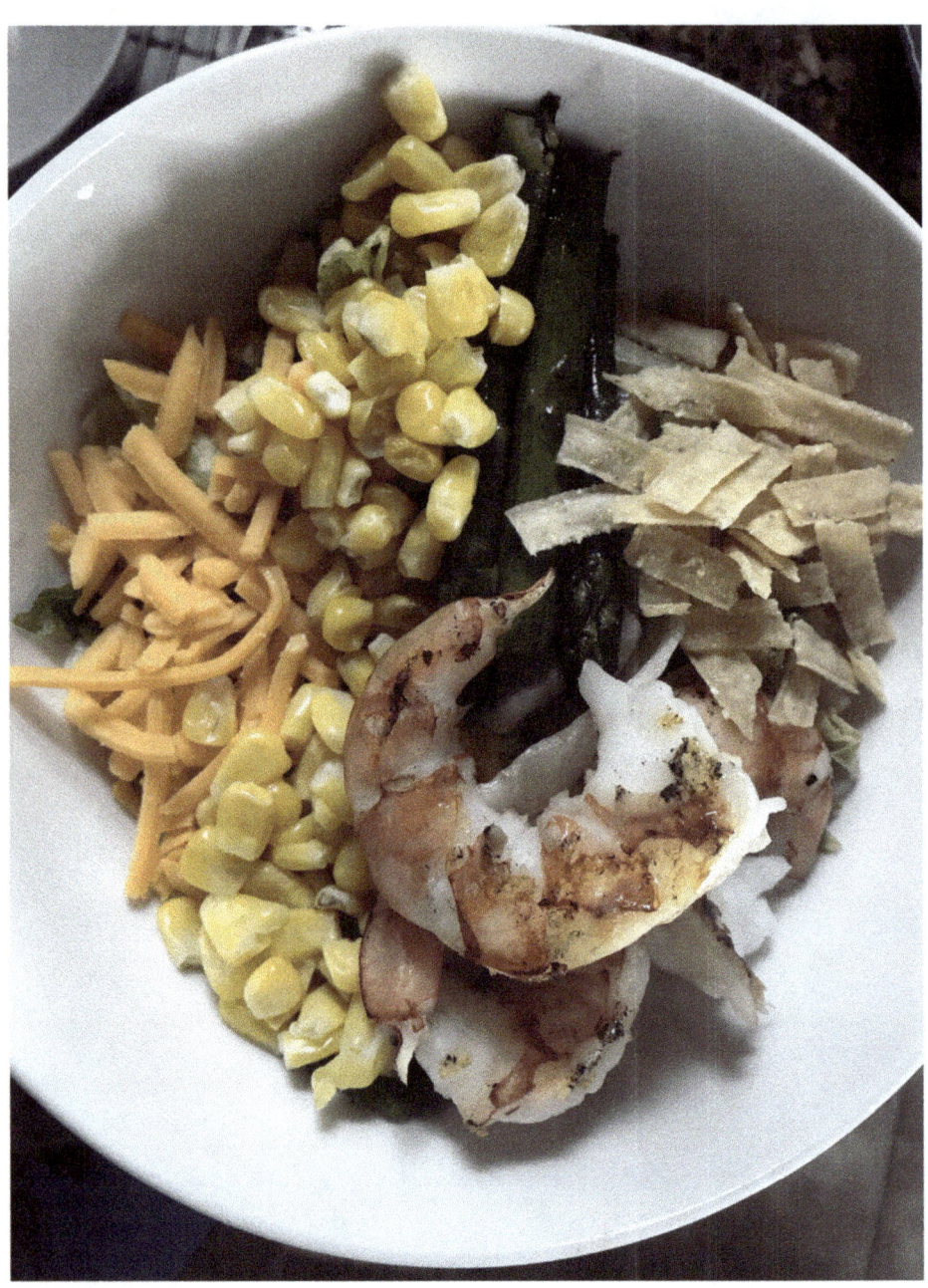

© copyright 2021 – all rights reserved.

the content contained within this book may not be reproduced, duplicated or transmitted without direct written permission from the author or the publisher.

under no circumstances will any blame or legal responsibility be held against the publisher, or author, for any damages, reparation, or monetary loss due to the information contained within this book. either directly or indirectly.

legal notice:

this book is copyright protected. this book is only for personal use. you cannot amend, distribute, sell, use, quote or paraphrase any part, or the content within this book, without the consent of the author or publisher.

disclaimer notice:

please note the information contained within this document is for educational and entertainment purposes only. all effort has been executed to present accurate, up to date, and reliable, complete information. no warranties of any kind are declared or implied. readers acknowledge that the author is not engaging in the rendering of legal, financial, medical or professional advice. the content within this book has been derived from various sources. please consult a licensed professional before attempting

any techniques outlined in this book.

by reading this document, the reader agrees that under no circumstances is the author responsible for any losses, direct or indirect, which are incurred as a result of the use of information contained within this document, including, but not limited to, — errors, omissions, or inaccuracies.

Table of Contents

SOUTHWEST SHRIMP 6

EASY SPICY SHRIMP 8

PERFECT AIR FRIED SHRIMP 10

HEALTHY COD FISH FILLETS 12

FLAVORFUL SALMON STEAK 14

HONEY GARLIC SHRIMP SKEWERS 17

FLAVORFUL SPICY SHRIMP 19

SCALLOPS WITH SAUCE 21

TASTY TUNA CAKES 23

EASY SALMON PATTIES 25

QUICK & EASY SCALLOPS 27

CAJUN SCALLOPS 30

CREAMY SCALLOPS 32

FLAVORS CRAB CAKES 34

QUICK & EASY SALMON PATTIES 36

HEALTHY SALMON PATTIES 38

CHEESY SALMON 40

TASTY PESTO SALMON 42

EVERYTHING BAGEL SALMON 44

PESTO WHITE FISH FILLETS 46

BAGEL CRUST WHITE FISH FILLETS 48

PARMESAN WHITE FISH FILLETS 50

HEALTHY MIX VEGETABLES 52

HEALTHY ASPARAGUS 55

GARLIC CHEESE BROCCOLI 57

SALT AND PEPPER SHRIMP 59

TUNA PATTIES 61

LEMON GARLIC SHRIMP	63
TASTY STEAMED LOBSTER TAILS	65
SPICY STEAMED SHRIMPS	67
WALLEYE PICKEREL WITH BUTTER AND LEMON	69
STEAMED TILAPIA AND VEGGIES	71
TASTY STEAMED FISH	74
CHINESE STYLE STEAMED GARLIC PRAWN	76
STEAMED LEMON GRASS CRAB LEGS	79
HEALTHY EGG BITES	81
EASY POTATO WEDGES	83
SWEET POTATOES & BRUSSELS SPROUTS	85
HEALTHY SPINACH FRITTATA	87
BREAKFAST POTATOES	90
SPINACH PEPPER EGG BITES	92
EGG CHEESE MUFFINS	94
MUSHROOM SPINACH MUFFINS	97
EGG VEGGIE SOUFFLÉ	99
ITALIAN EGG MUFFINS	101
MARINATED GINGER GARLIC SALMON	103

Southwest Shrimp

Preparation Time: 10 minutes

Cooking Time: 6 minutes

Serve: 4

Nutritional Value (Amount per Serving):

- Calories 143
- Fat 2.9 g
- Carbohydrates 1.7 g
- Sugar 0 g
- Protein 25.8 g
- Cholesterol 241 mg

Ingredients:

- 1 lb shrimp, peeled & deveined
- 1 1/2 tsp southwestern seasoning
- 1 tsp butter, melted

Directions:

1. In a bowl, toss shrimp with seasoning and melted butter.
2. Preheat the air fryer to 400 F.
3. Add shrimp into the air fryer basket and cook for 6 minutes.
4. Serve and enjoy.

Easy Spicy Shrimp

Preparation Time: 10 minutes

Cooking Time: 7 minutes

Serve: 4

Nutritional Value (Amount per Serving):

- Calories 150
- Fat 3.4 g
- Carbohydrates 2.7 g
- Sugar 0.1 g
- Protein 26.1 g
- Cholesterol 239 mg

Ingredients:

- 1 lb shrimp
- 1/4 tsp ground mustard
- 1/4 tsp ground cumin

- 1/4 tsp oregano
- 1/4 tsp thyme
- 1/4 tsp cayenne
- 1/4 tsp garlic powder
- 1/2 tsp paprika
- 1 tsp chili powder
- 1 tsp olive oil
- Pepper
- Salt

Directions:

1. Preheat the air fryer to 400 F.
2. Add shrimp and remaining ingredients into the bowl and toss well.
3. Add shrimp mixture into the air fryer basket and cook for 7 minutes. Stir halfway through.
4. Serve and enjoy.

Perfect Air Fried Shrimp

Preparation Time: 10 minutes

Cooking Time: 8 minutes

Serve: 4

Nutritional Value (Amount per Serving):

- Calories 158
- Fat 4.4 g
- Carbohydrates 2.1 g
- Sugar 0.2 g
- Protein 25.9 g
- Cholesterol 239 mg

Ingredients:

- 1 lb shrimp
- 1/2 tsp Italian seasoning
- 1/4 tsp paprika

- 1/2 tsp garlic powder
- 2 tsp olive oil
- Pepper
- Salt

Directions:

1. Preheat the air fryer to 400 F.
2. Add shrimp and remaining ingredients into the bowl and toss well.
3. Add shrimp mixture into the air fryer basket and cook for 8 minutes.
4. Serve and enjoy.

Healthy Cod Fish Fillets

Preparation Time: 10 minutes

Cooking Time: 10 minutes

Serve: 4

Nutritional Value (Amount per Serving):

- Calories 64
- Fat 2.3 g
- Carbohydrates 7 g
- Sugar 0.4 g
- Protein 3.8 g
- Cholesterol 82 mg

Ingredients:

- 2 eggs
- 1 tsp garlic powder
- 1 tsp lemon pepper seasoning

- 1 cup parmesan cheese, grated
- 1 cup almond flour
- 1/2 cup whole-wheat breadcrumbs
- 1/4 cup all-purpose flour
- 4 cod fillets
- Pepper
- Salt

Directions:

1. In a small bowl, whisk eggs with pepper and salt.
2. In a shallow dish, mix breadcrumbs, almond flour, cheese, lemon pepper seasoning, and garlic powder.
3. In a separate bowl, add flour.
4. Coat fish fillets with flour then dip in the egg mixture and finally coat with breadcrumb mixture.
5. Place coated fish fillets into the air fryer basket and cook at 350 F for 8-10 minutes.
6. Serve and enjoy.

Flavorful Salmon Steak

Preparation Time: 10 minutes

Cooking Time: 14 minutes

Serve: 2

Nutritional Value (Amount per Serving):

- Calories 441
- Fat 34.1 g
- Carbohydrates 0.5 g
- Sugar 0 g
- Protein 34.9 g
- Cholesterol 140 mg

Ingredients:

- 2 salmon steaks
- 2 tsp ground sage
- 4 tbsp butter, melted

- Pepper
- Salt

Directions:

1. In a small bowl, mix butter, sage, pepper, and salt.
2. Brush salmon steaks with butter mixture and place into the air fryer basket and cook at 400 F for 14 minutes.
3. Serve and enjoy.

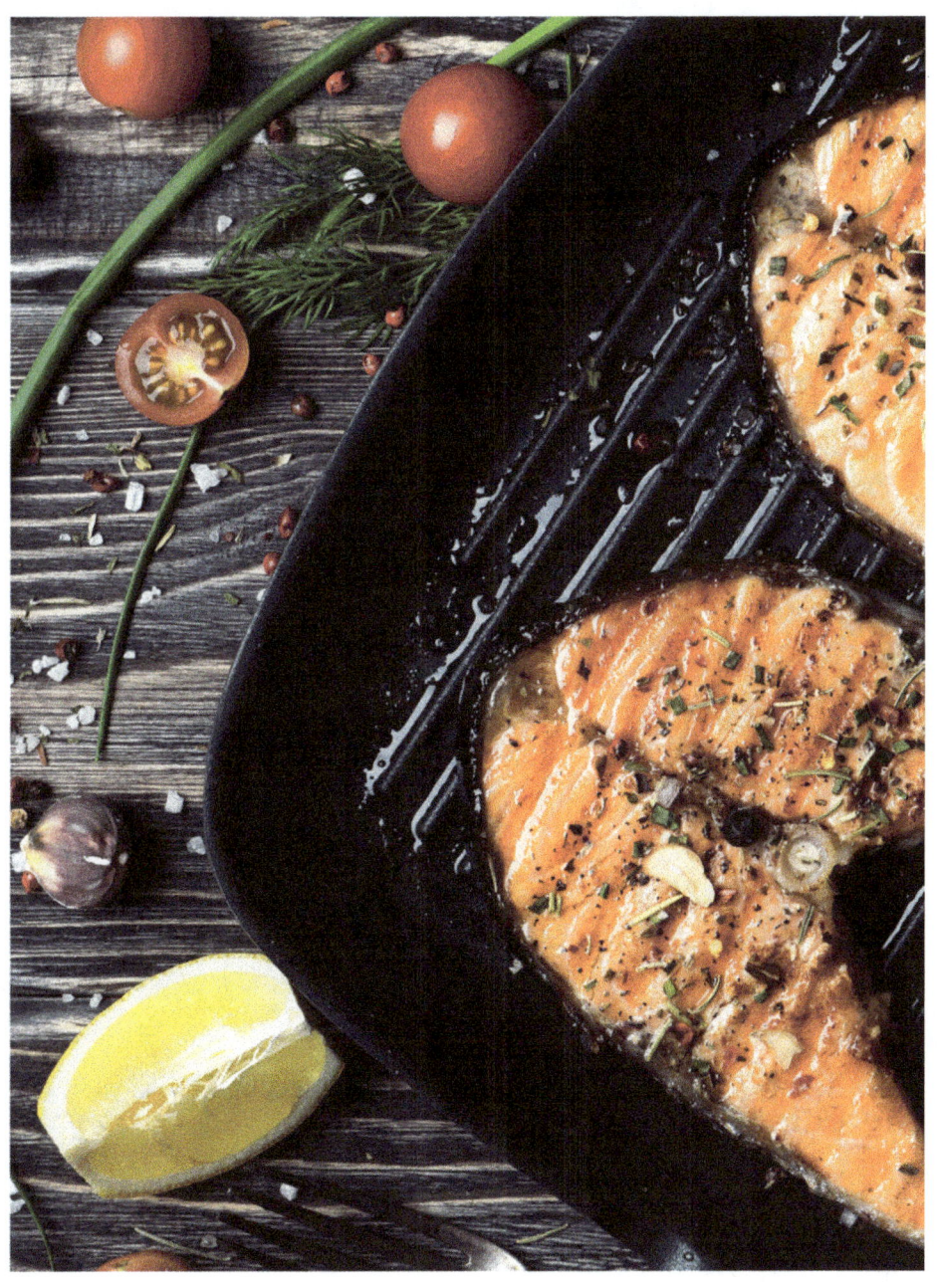

Honey Garlic Shrimp Skewers

Preparation Time: 10 minutes

Cooking Time: 5 minutes

Serve: 4

Nutritional Value (Amount per Serving):

- Calories 332
- Fat 8.9 g
- Carbohydrates 38 g
- Sugar 35 g
- Protein 26.8 g
- Cholesterol 239 mg

Ingredients:

- 1 lb shrimp
- 2 tsp garlic, minced
- 2 tbsp olive oil

- 3 tbsp soy sauce
- 1/2 cup honey

Directions:

1. Add shrimp, garlic, oil, soy sauce, and honey into the bowl and mix well. Cover and place in the refrigerator for overnight.
2. Thread marinated shrimp onto the soaked wooden skewers.
3. Place shrimp skewers into the air fryer basket and cook at 400 F for 5 minutes.
4. Serve and enjoy.

Flavorful Spicy Shrimp

Preparation Time: 10 minutes

Cooking Time: 10 minutes

Serve: 4

Nutritional Value (Amount per Serving):

- Calories 287
- Fat 4.2 g
- Carbohydrates 6.6 g
- Sugar 1.5 g
- Protein 52.6 g
- Cholesterol 478 mg

Ingredients:

- 2 lb shrimp, peeled & deveined
- 1 tbsp lemon juice
- 2 tbsp soy sauce

- 1 tsp garlic powder
- 1 tsp sugar
- 1 tsp ground cumin
- 1 tsp liquid smoke
- 1 tsp chili powder
- 1 tbsp Tabasco sauce
- 1 tsp paprika
- Pepper
- Salt

Directions:

1. Add shrimp and remaining ingredients into the bowl and toss well.
2. Add shrimp mixture into the air fryer basket and cook at 400 F for 10 minutes. Stir halfway through.
3. Serve and enjoy.

Scallops with Sauce

Preparation Time: 10 minutes

Cooking Time: 7 minutes

Serve: 4

Nutritional Value (Amount per Serving):

- Calories 238
- Fat 15 g
- Carbohydrates 4.5 g
- Sugar 1 g
- Protein 20.9 g
- Cholesterol 57 mg

Ingredients:

- 1 lb sea scallops
- 2 tsp garlic, minced
- 3 tbsp heavy cream

- 1/4 cup pesto
- 1 tbsp olive oil
- Pepper
- Salt

Directions:

1. Season scallops with pepper and salt.
2. Place scallops into the air fryer basket and cook at 320 F for 5 minutes.
3. In a pan, add cream, pesto, oil, and garlic and cook for 2 minutes.
4. Pour sauce over cooked scallops and serve.

Tasty Tuna Cakes

Preparation Time: 10 minutes

Cooking Time: 6 minutes

Serve: 4

Nutritional Value (Amount per Serving):

- Calories 113
- Fat 2.7 g
- Carbohydrates 5.9 g
- Sugar 0.7 g
- Protein 15.6 g
- Cholesterol 56 mg

Ingredients:

- 1 egg
- 7 oz can tuna
- 1/4 cup whole-wheat breadcrumbs

- 1 tbsp mustard
- Pepper
- Salt

Directions:

1. Add all ingredients into the bowl and mix until well combined.
2. Make patties from the mixture and place into the air fryer basket and cook at 400 F for 6 minutes. Turn patties halfway through.
3. Serve and enjoy.

Easy Salmon Patties

Preparation Time: 10 minutes

Cooking Time: 10 minutes

Serve: 4

Nutritional Value (Amount per Serving):

- Calories 157
- Fat 7.1 g
- Carbohydrates 0.9 g
- Sugar 0.4 g
- Protein 21.1 g
- Cholesterol 95 mg

Ingredients:

- 1 egg
- 1 tsp dill weed
- 1/2 cup whole-wheat breadcrumbs

- 1/4 cup onion, chopped
- 14 oz can salmon, remove bones & skin
- Pepper
- Salt

Directions:

1. Add all ingredients into the bowl and mix until well combined.
2. Make patties from the mixture and place into the air fryer basket and cook at 370 F for 10 minutes. Turn patties halfway through.
3. Serve and enjoy.

Quick & Easy Scallops

Preparation Time: 10 minutes

Cooking Time: 4 minutes

Serve: 2

Nutritional Value (Amount per Serving):

- Calories 126
- Fat 3.2 g
- Carbohydrates 2.9 g
- Sugar 0 g
- Protein 20.2 g
- Cholesterol 40 mg

Ingredients:

- 8 scallops
- 1 tsp olive oil
- Pepper

- Salt

Directions:

1. Preheat the air fryer to 390 F.
2. Add scallops, oil, pepper, and salt into the bowl and toss well.
3. Add scallops into the air fryer basket and cook for 4 minutes. Turn scallops halfway through.
4. Serve and enjoy.

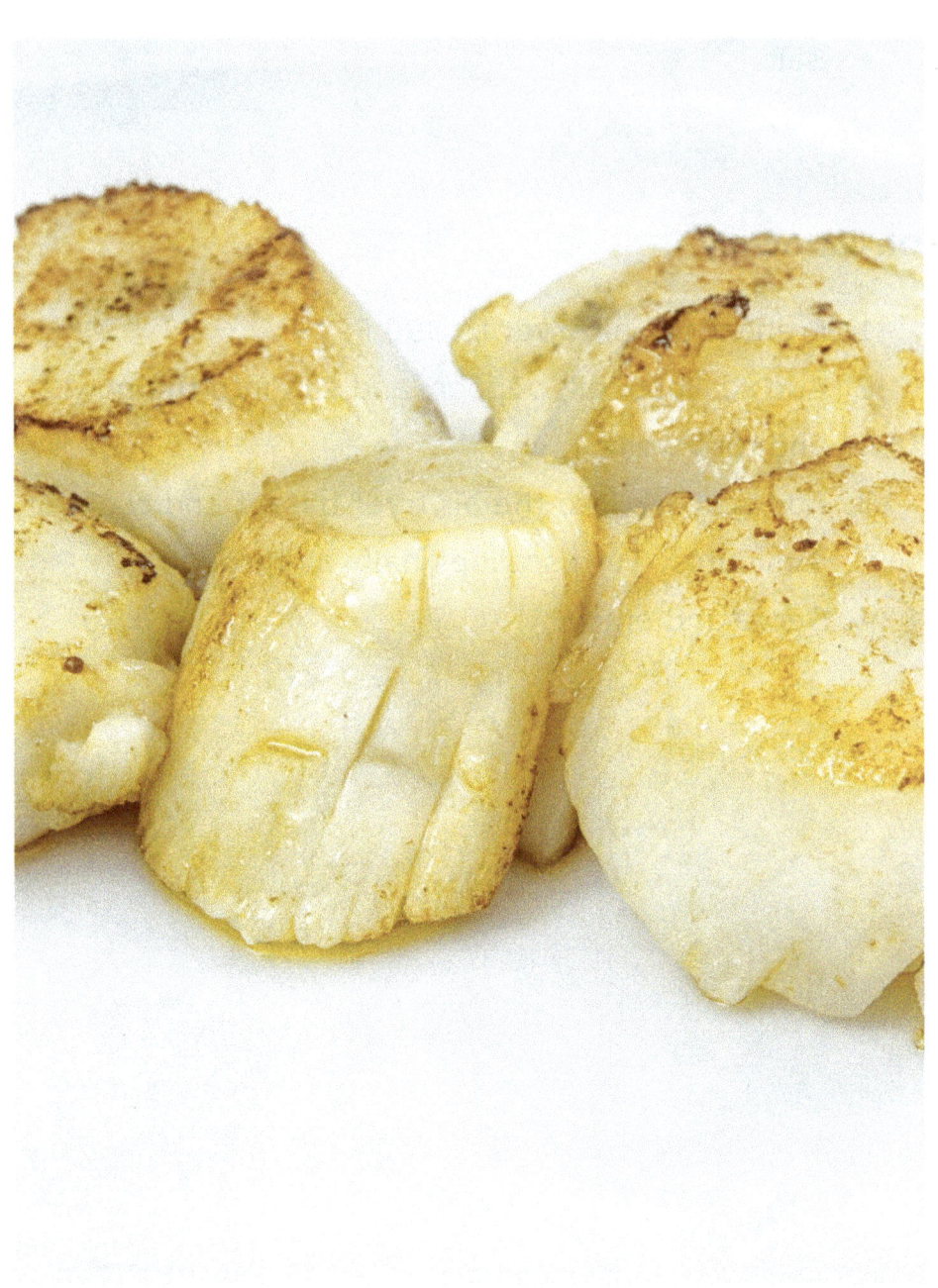

Cajun Scallops

Preparation Time: 10 minutes

Cooking Time: 6 minutes

Serve: 2

Nutritional Value (Amount per Serving):

- Calories 99
- Fat 3 g
- Carbohydrates 2.1 g
- Sugar 0 g
- Protein 15.1 g
- Cholesterol 30 mg

Ingredients:

- 6 scallops
- 1/2 tsp Cajun seasoning
- 1 tsp olive oil

- Salt

Directions:

1. Preheat the air fryer to 400 F.
2. Add scallops, oil, Cajun seasoning, and salt into the bowl and toss well.
3. Add scallops into the air fryer basket and cook for 6 minutes. Turn scallops halfway through.
4. Serve and enjoy.

Creamy Scallops

Preparation Time: 10 minutes

Cooking Time: 10 minutes

Serve: 4

Nutritional Value (Amount per Serving):

- Calories 220
- Fat 13.7 g
- Carbohydrates 3.4 g
- Sugar 0.1 g
- Protein 19.4 g
- Cholesterol 76 mg

Ingredients:

- 1 lb sea scallops
- 1 tbsp white wine
- 1 tsp garlic, minced

- 2 tsp lemon juice
- 3 tbsp heavy cream
- 3 tbsp butter
- Pepper
- Salt

Directions:

1. Preheat the air fryer to 400 F.
2. Season scallops with pepper and salt and place into the air fryer basket and cook for 10 minutes. Turn scallops halfway through.
3. Melt butter in a pan over medium heat.
4. Add garlic and sauté for 30 seconds. Add wine, lemon juice, and heavy cream and stir until thickened.
5. Pour sauce over cooked scallops and serve.

Flavors Crab Cakes

Preparation Time: 10 minutes

Cooking Time: 12 minutes

Serve: 4

Nutritional Value (Amount per Serving):

- Calories 187
- Fat 8.3 g
- Carbohydrates 8 g
- Sugar 2.1 g
- Protein 16.5 g
- Cholesterol 105 mg

Ingredients:

- 1 egg
- 1 lb crab meat
- 1 tbsp capers
- 1 roasted red pepper, diced
- 2 green onions, chopped

- 2/3 cup whole-wheat breadcrumbs
- 1 tbsp parsley, chopped
- 1/2 lemon juice
- 2 tsp old bay seasoning
- 1 tbsp soy sauce
- 1 tbsp Dijon mustard
- 1/4 cup mayonnaise
- Salt

Directions:

1. Preheat the air fryer to 360 F.
2. Spray air fryer basket with cooking spray.
3. Add all ingredients into the mixing bowl and mix until well combined.
4. Make the equal shape of patties from the mixture and place into the air fryer basket and cook for 7 minutes.
5. Flip patties and cook for 5 minutes more.
6. Serve and enjoy.

Quick & Easy Salmon Patties

Preparation Time: 10 minutes

Cooking Time: 8 minutes

Serve: 6

Nutritional Value (Amount per Serving):

- Calories 105
- Fat 4.8 g
- Carbohydrates 0.6 g
- Sugar 0.2 g
- Protein 14.2 g
- Cholesterol 64 mg

Ingredients:

- 1 egg
- 1 tsp paprika
- 2 green onions, minced

- 2 tbsp fresh coriander, chopped
- 14 oz can salmon, drain & remove bones Salt

Directions:

1. Preheat the air fryer to 360 F.
2. Add all ingredients into the mixing bowl and mix until well combined.
3. Make the equal shape of patties from the mixture and place into the air fryer basket and cook for 8 minutes.
4. Serve and enjoy.

Healthy Salmon Patties

Preparation Time: 10 minutes

Cooking Time: 15 minutes

Serve: 4

Nutritional Value (Amount per Serving):

- Calories 60
- Fat 3.2 g
- Carbohydrates 1.9 g
- Sugar 0.5 g
- Protein 6.4 g
- Cholesterol 88 mg

Ingredients:

- 2 eggs, lightly beaten
- 2 oz salmon, cooked & flaked

- 2 tsp nutritional yeast
- 1/4 tsp paprika
- 1 tsp garlic, minced
- 1/4 cup onion, diced
- 2/3 cup almond flour
- Pepper
- Salt

Directions:

1. Preheat the air fryer to 380 F.
2. Add all ingredients into the mixing bowl and mix until well combined.
3. Make the equal shape of patties from the mixture and place into the air fryer basket and cook for 12-15 minutes.
4. Serve and enjoy.

Cheesy Salmon

Preparation Time: 10 minutes

Cooking Time: 7 minutes

Serve: 4

Nutritional Value (Amount per Serving):

- Calories 279
- Fat 14.7 g
- Carbohydrates 2.7 g
- Sugar 0.7 g
- Protein 34.6 g
- Cholesterol 81 mg

Ingredients:

- 4 salmon fillets
- 1/4 cup parmesan cheese, grated
- 3 tbsp mayonnaise

- Pepper
- Salt

Directions:

1. Preheat the air fryer to 400 F.
2. Spray air fryer basket with cooking spray.
3. In a bowl, mix cheese, mayonnaise, pepper, and salt.
4. Spread cheese mixture on top of fish fillets.
5. Place fish fillets into the air fryer basket and cook for 7 minutes.
6. Serve and enjoy.

Tasty Pesto Salmon

Preparation Time: 10 minutes

Cooking Time: 15 minutes

Serve: 4

Nutritional Value (Amount per Serving):

- Calories 333
- Fat 21 g
- Carbohydrates 1 g
- Sugar 1 g
- Protein 36 g
- Cholesterol 82 mg

Ingredients:

- 4 salmon fillets
- 1 tbsp olive oil
- 1/4 cup pesto

Directions:

1. Preheat the air fryer to 360 F.
2. Spray air fryer basket with cooking spray.
3. Place salmon fillets into the air fryer basket. Mix pesto and oil and spread on top of salmon fillets.
4. Cook salmon fillets for 12-15 minutes.
5. Serve and enjoy.

Everything Bagel Salmon

Preparation Time: 10 minutes

Cooking Time: 12 minutes

Serve: 2

Nutritional Value (Amount per Serving):

- Calories 355
- Fat 25 g
- Carbohydrates 0 g
- Sugar 0 g
- Protein 34.5 g
- Cholesterol 78 mg

Ingredients:

- 2 salmon fillets
- 4 tbsp everything bagel seasoning
- 2 tbsp olive oil

Directions:

1. Preheat the air fryer to 350 F.
2. Spray air fryer basket with cooking spray.
3. Brush salmon fillets with oil and coat with bagel seasoning.
4. Place fish fillets into the air fryer basket and cook for 12 minutes.
5. Serve and enjoy.

Pesto White Fish Fillets

Preparation Time: 10 minutes

Cooking Time: 8 minutes

Serve: 2

Nutritional Value (Amount per Serving):

- Calories 326
- Fat 18.6 g
- Carbohydrates 0.1 g
- Sugar 0 g
- Protein 37.8 g
- Cholesterol 119 mg

Ingredients:

- 2 white fish fillets
- 1 tbsp olive oil
- 1/4 cup basil pesto

Directions:

1. Preheat the air fryer to 360 F.
2. Spray air fryer basket with cooking spray.
3. Place fish fillets into the air fryer basket. Mix pesto and oil and spread on top of fish fillets.
4. Cook fish fillets for 8 minutes.
5. Serve and enjoy.

Bagel Crust White Fish Fillets

Preparation Time: 10 minutes

Cooking Time: 10 minutes

Serve: 4

Nutritional Value (Amount per Serving):

- Calories 281
- Fat 12.8 g
- Carbohydrates 1.2 g
- Sugar 0.2 g
- Protein 37.8 g
- Cholesterol 120 mg

Ingredients:

- 4 white fish fillets
- 1 tbsp mayonnaise
- 1 tsp lemon pepper seasoning

- 2 tbsp almond flour
- 4 tbsp everything bagel seasoning

Directions:

1. Preheat the air fryer to 375 F.
2. In a shallow dish, mix almond flour, lemon pepper seasoning, and bagel seasoning.
3. Brush fish fillets with mayonnaise and coat with almond flour mixture.
4. Place fish fillets into the air fryer basket and cook for 8-10 minutes.
5. Serve and enjoy.

Parmesan White Fish Fillets

Preparation Time: 10 minutes

Cooking Time: 15 minutes

Serve: 2

Nutritional Value (Amount per Serving):

- Calories 331
- Fat 18.7 g
- Carbohydrates 1.3 g
- Sugar 0.4 g
- Protein 38 g
- Cholesterol 119 mg

Ingredients:

- 2 white fish fillets
- 1/2 tsp paprika
- 1/2 tsp onion powder

- 1/2 tsp garlic powder
- 1/2 cup parmesan cheese, grated
- 1 tbsp olive oil
- Pepper
- Salt

Directions:

1. Preheat the air fryer to 380 F.
2. In a shallow dish, mix cheese, garlic powder, onion powder, paprika, pepper, and salt.
3. Brush fish fillets with oil and coat with cheese mixture.
4. Spray air fryer basket with cooking spray.
5. Place coated fish fillets into the air fryer basket and cook for 12-15 minutes.
6. Serve and enjoy.

Healthy Mix Vegetables

Preparation Time: 10 minutes

Cooking Time: 18 minutes

Serve: 4

Nutritional Value (Amount per Serving):

- Calories 56
- Fat 3.6 g
- Carbohydrates 5.6 g
- Sugar 2.3 g
- Protein 1.4 g
- Cholesterol 0 mg

Ingredients:

- 1 cup broccoli florets
- 1 cup carrots, sliced
- 1 cup cauliflower, cut into florets

- ¼ tsp garlic powder
- 1 tbsp olive oil
- Pepper
- Salt

Directions:

1. Add all ingredients into the bowl and toss well.
2. Add vegetable mixture into the air fryer basket and cook at 380 F for 18 minutes. Stir halfway through.
3. Serve and enjoy.

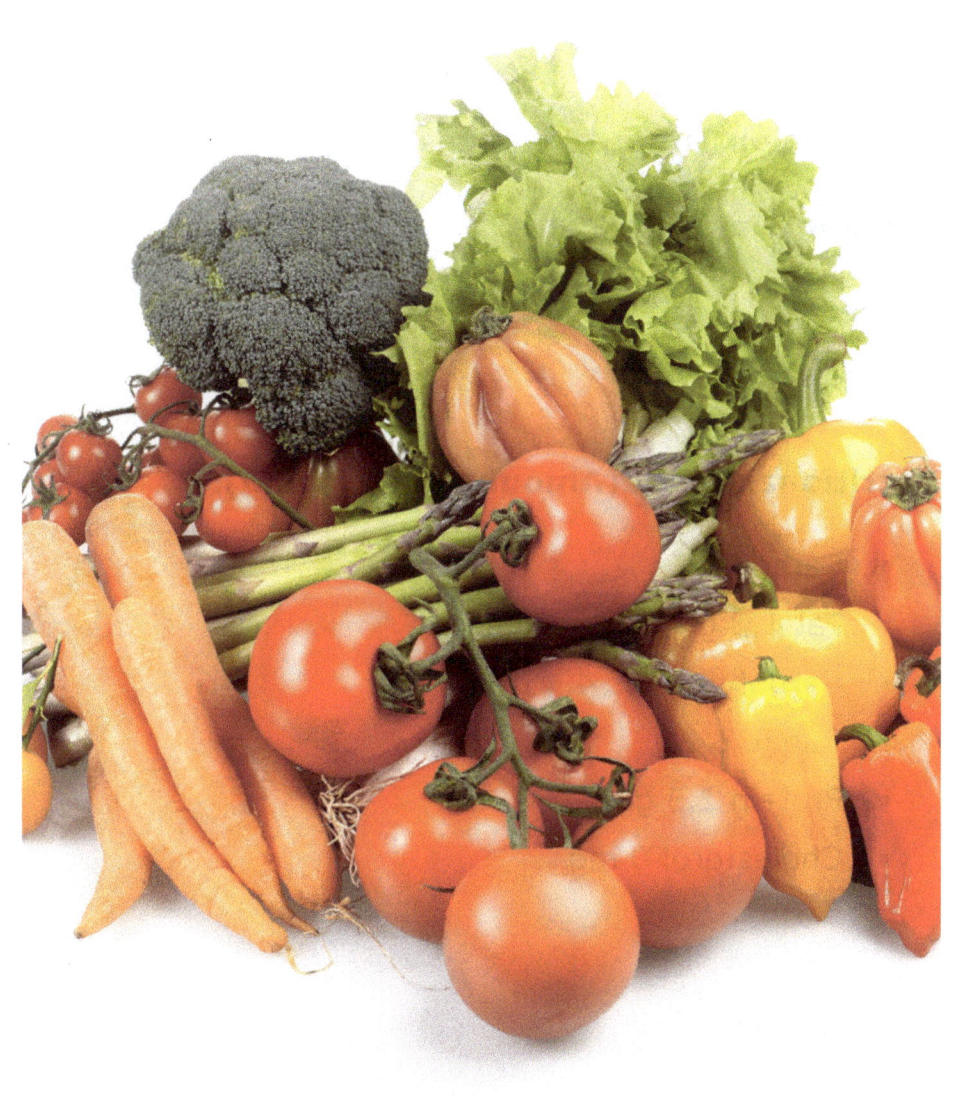

Healthy Asparagus

Preparation Time: 10 minutes

Cooking Time: 7 minutes

Serve: 4

Nutritional Value (Amount per Serving):

- Calories 35
- Fat 1.3 g
- Carbohydrates 4.4 g
- Sugar 2.1 g
- Protein 2.5 g
- Cholesterol 0 mg

Ingredients:

- 1 lb asparagus, cut the ends
- 1 tsp butter, melted
- Pepper

- Salt

Directions:

1. Preheat the air fryer to 350 F.
2. Add asparagus, butter, pepper, and salt into the bowl and toss well.
3. Add asparagus into the air fryer basket and cook for 7 minutes.
4. Serve and enjoy.

Garlic Cheese Broccoli

Preparation Time: 10 minutes

Cooking Time: 5 minutes

Serve: 4

Nutritional Value (Amount per Serving):

- Calories 250
- Fat 16.4 g
- Carbohydrates 8.2 g
- Sugar 2 g

- Protein 15.3 g
- Cholesterol 30 mg

Ingredients:

- 1 lb broccoli florets
- 2 tbsp butter, melted

- ¼ tsp chili flakes, crushed
- ¼ cup parmesan cheese, grated
- 1 tbsp garlic, minced
- Pepper
- Salt

Directions:

1. Preheat the air fryer to 350 F.
2. Add broccoli and remaining ingredients into the bowl and toss well.
3. Add broccoli mixture into the air fryer basket and cook for 5 minutes.
4. Serve and enjoy.

Salt and Pepper Shrimp

Servings: 4

Total Time: 30 Minutes

Calories: 228

Fat: 8.9 g

Protein: 26.4 g

Carbs: 9.3 g

Ingredients and Quantity

- 2 tsp. peppercorns
- 1 tsp. salt
- 1 tsp. sugar
- 1 lb. shrimp
- 3 tbsp. rice flour
- 2 tbsp. oil

Direction

1. Set the Foodi to sauté.
2. Roast the peppercorns for 1 minute and then allow them cool.
3. Crush the peppercorns and add the salt and sugar.
4. Coat the shrimp with this mixture and then with flour.
5. Sprinkle oil on the Ninja Foodi basket.
6. Place the shrimp on top.
7. Cook at 350 degrees for 10 minutes, flipping halfway through.
8. You can serve with fresh salad. Enjoy!

Tuna Patties

Servings: 2

Total Time: 45 Minutes

Calories: 141

Fat: 6.4 g

Protein: 17 g

Carbs: 5.2 g

Ingredients and Quantity

- 2 cans tuna flakes
- 1/2 tbsp. almond flour
- 1 tsp. dried dill
- 1 tbsp. vegan mayo
- 1/2 tsp. onion powder
- tsp. garlic powder
- Salt and pepper, to taste
- 1 tbsp. lemon juice

Direction

1. Mix all the ingredients in a bowl and then form patties.
2. Set the tuna patties on the Ninja Foodi basket.
3. Seal the crisping lid.
4. Set it to air crisp.
5. Cook at 400 degrees for 10 minutes.
6. Flip and cook for 5 more minutes.
7. You can serve with fresh green salad. Enjoy!

Lemon Garlic Shrimp

Servings: 4

Total Time: 50 Minutes

Calories: 170

Fat: 5.5 g

Protein: 26.1 g

Carbs: 2.8 g

Ingredients and Quantity

- 1 lb. shrimp, peeled and deveined
- 1 tbsp. olive oil
- 4 garlic cloves, minced
- 1 tbsp. lemon juice
- Salt, to taste

Direction

1. Mix the olive oil, salt, lemon juice and garlic.

2. Toss shrimp in the mixture.

3. Marinate for 15 minutes.

4. Place the shrimp in the Ninja Foodi basket.

5. Seal the crisping lid.

6. Select the air crisp setting.

7. Cook at 350 degrees for 8 minutes.

8. Flip and cook for 2 more minutes.

9. You can sprinkle chopped parsley on top. Enjoy!

Tasty Steamed Lobster Tails

Servings: 4

Total Time: 15 Minutes

Calories: 353

Fat: 24.5 g

Protein: 32.2 g

Carbs: 0.9 g

Ingredients and Quantity

- Four 6 oz. lobster tails
- Salt and pepper, to taste
- 1/2 cup butter

Direction

1. Place the Ninja Foodi reversible rack inside the ceramic pot.

2. Pour a cup of water in the pot.
3. Season the lobster tails with salt and pepper to taste.
4. Place the seasoned lobster tails on the reversible rack.
5. Close the pressure lid and set the vent to SEAL.
6. Press the Steam button and adjust cooking time to 10 minutes.
7. Do quick pressure release.
8. Once the lid is open, take the lobster tail out and serve with butter on top.

Spicy Steamed Shrimps

Servings: 2

Total Time: 12 Minutes

Calories: 360

Fat: 4.4 g

Protein: 41.1 g

Carbs: 38.8 g

Ingredients and Quantity

- 1 pound tiger prawns with shell
- 1 packet Old Bay seasoning
- 1 jar cocktail sauce

Direction

1. Place the Ninja Foodi Cook and Crisp reversible rack inside the ceramic pot.

2. Pour a cup of water in the pot.

3. Season the prawns with Old Bay seasoning.

4. Place the shrimps on the reversible rack.

5. Close the pressure lid and set the vent to SEAL.

6. Press the Steam button and adjust the cooking time to 10 minutes.

7. Do quick pressure release.

8. Serve with cocktail sauce. Enjoy!

Walleye Pickerel with Butter and Lemon

Servings: 8

Total Time: 24 Minutes

Calories: 336

Fat: 15.6 g

Protein: 43.9 g

Carbs: 4.8 g

Ingredients and Quantity

- 8 fillets walleye pickerel
- 1/4 cup almond butter
- 1/4 cup lemon juice
- 1 large onion, sliced into rings
- Salt and pepper, to taste

Direction

1. Place the Foodi Cook and Crisp reversible rack inside the ceramic pot.
2. Pour a cup of water in the pot.
3. On a large aluminum foil, place the pickerel and pour over the almond butter, lemon juice, salt and pepper.
4. Garnish with onion rings on top.
5. Close the aluminum foil and crimp the edges.
6. Place on the reversible rack.
7. Close the pressure lid and set the vent to Seal.
8. Press the Steam button and adjust the cooking time to 20 minutes. Serve and enjoy!

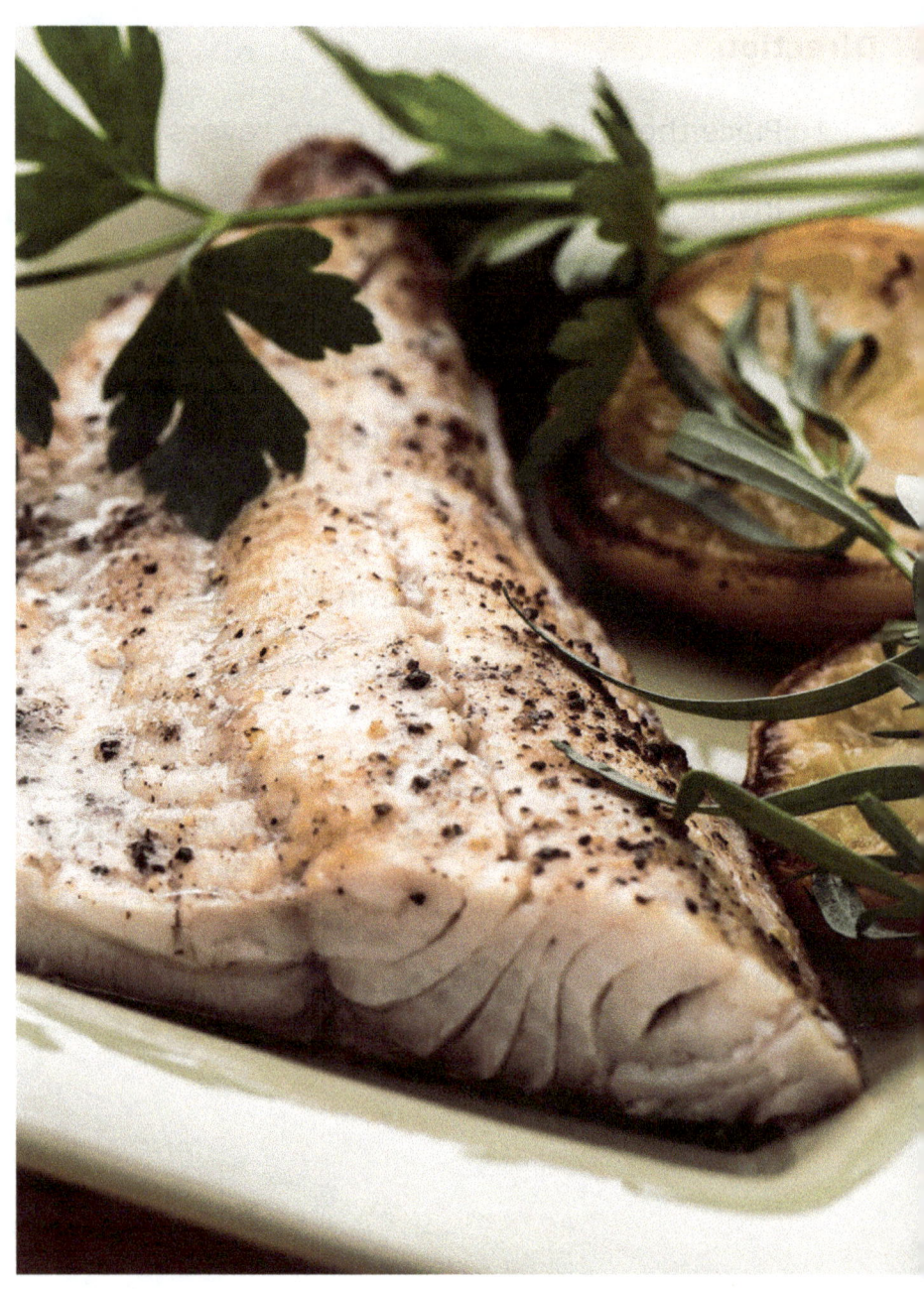

Steamed Tilapia and Veggies

Servings: 6

Total Time: 18 Minutes

Calories: 134

Fat: 2.4 g

Protein: 23.6 g

Carbs: 4.4 g

Ingredients and Quantity

- 1 tsp. olive oil
- 6 tilapia fillets
- 1 pinch Greek seasoning
- 4 stalks celery, halved
- 1 cup fresh baby carrots
- 1 bell pepper, cut into chunks
- 1/2 onion, sliced
- Salt and pepper, to taste

Direction

1. Place the Foodi Cook and Crisp reversible rack inside the ceramic pot.
2. Pour water into the pot.
3. Brush oil on to the tilapia fillets.
4. Season with Greek seasoning, salt and pepper.
5. Place the tilapia fillets on the basket.
6. Layer the veggies on top.
7. Close the pressure lid and set the vent to Seal.
8. Press the Steam button and adjust the cooking time to 15 minutes. Serve and enjoy!

Tasty Steamed Fish

Servings: 6

Total Time: 18 Minutes

Calories: 137

Fat: 1.1 g

Protein: 29.7 g

Carbs: 1.9 g

Ingredients and Quantity

- 6 halibut fillets
- 1 tbsp. dried dill weed
- 1 tbsp. onion powder
- 2 tsp. dried parsley
- 1/4 tsp. paprika
- 1 pinch salt
- 1 pinch lemon pepper
- 1 pinch garlic powder

- 2 tbsp. lemon juice

Direction

1. Place the Ninja Foodi Cook and Crisp reversible rack inside the ceramic pot.
2. Pour water into the pot.
3. Season the halibut fillets with dill weed, onion powder, dried parsley, paprika, salt, pepper, garlic powder, and lemon juice.
4. Place the seasoned fish fillets on the reversible rack.
5. Close the pressure lid and set the vent to SEAL.
6. Press the Steam button and adjust the cooking time to 15 minutes. Serve and enjoy!

Chinese Style Steamed Garlic Prawn

Servings: 10

Total Time: 25 Minutes

Calories: 67

Fat: 1.8 g

Protein: 12.1 g

Carbs: 1.8 g

Ingredients and Quantity

- 20 large tiger prawns, shells not removed
- 2 tbsp. soy sauce
- 5 garlic cloves, minced
- 1 tbsp. brandy

Direction

1. Place all ingredients in a Ziploc bag and marinate in the fridge for at least 2 hours.
2. Place the Foodi Cook and Crisp reversible rack inside the ceramic pot.
3. Pour water into the pot.
4. Place the marinated shrimps on the reversible rack.
5. Close the pressure lid and set the vent to SEAL.
6. Press the Steam button and adjust the cooking time to 20 minutes. Serve and enjoy!

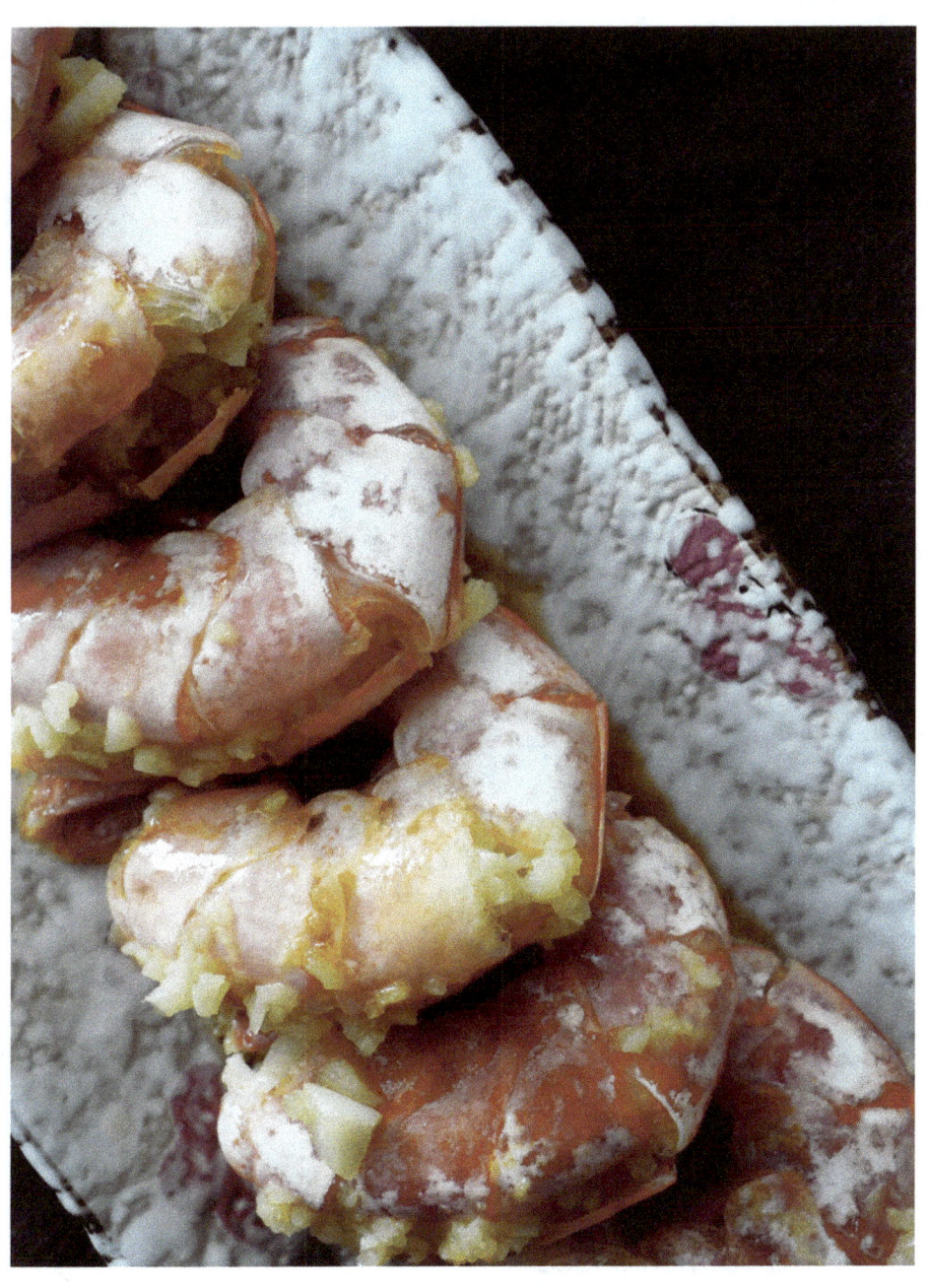

Steamed Lemon Grass Crab Legs

Servings: 4

Total Time: 30 Minutes

Calories: 564

Fat: 20.7 g

Protein: 89.1 g

Carbs: 5.3 g

Ingredients and Quantity

- 2 tbsp. vegetable oil
- 3 garlic cloves, minced
- 1 piece fresh ginger root, crushed
- 1 stalk lemon grass, crushed
- 2 tbsp. fish sauce
- 1 tbsp. oyster sauce

- 2 pounds frozen Alaskan king crab
- Salt and pepper, to taste

Direction

1. Place the Foodi Cook and Crisp reversible rack inside the ceramic pot.
2. Pour water into the pot.
3. Combine all ingredients in a big Ziploc bag and marinate for at least 30 minutes.
4. Place the crabs on the reversible rack.
5. Close the pressure lid and set the vent to Seal.
6. Press the Steam button and adjust the cooking time to 25 minutes. Serve and enjoy!

Healthy Egg Bites

Preparation Time: 10 minutes

Cooking Time: 13 minutes

Serve: 4

Nutritional Value (Amount per Serving):

- Calories 125
- Fat 8.1 g
- Carbohydrates 2.8 g
- Sugar 2.1 g
- Protein 9.8 g
- Cholesterol 178 mg

Ingredients:

- 4 eggs, lightly beaten
- ¼ cup cheddar cheese, shredded
- ½ cup bell pepper, diced

- ½ cup almond milk
- ¼ tsp garlic powder
- Pepper
- Salt

Directions:

1. Preheat the air fryer to 325 F.
2. Add all ingredients into the bowl and whisk until well combined.
3. Spray silicone muffin molds with cooking spray.
4. Pour egg mixture into the silicone muffin mold and place it in the air fryer basket and cook for 8-10 minutes.
5. Serve and enjoy.

Easy Potato Wedges

Preparation Time: 10 minutes

Cooking Time: 10 minutes

Serve: 6

Nutritional Value (Amount per Serving):

- Calories 174
- Fat 8.6 g
- Carbohydrates 23.8 g
- Sugar 1.7 g
- Protein 2.5 g
- Cholesterol 0 mg

Ingredients:

- 2 lbs potatoes, cut into wedges
- 2 tbsp chipotle seasoning
- ¼ cup olive oil

- Pepper
- Salt

Directions:

1. Add potato wedges into the bowl.
2. Add remaining ingredients over potato wedges and toss well.
3. Transfer potato wedges into the air fryer basket and cook for 10 minutes. Turn potato wedges halfway through.
4. Serve and enjoy.

Sweet Potatoes & Brussels Sprouts

Preparation Time: 10 minutes

Cooking Time: 20 minutes

Serve: 4

Nutritional Value (Amount per Serving):

- Calories 135
- Fat 7.4 g
- Carbohydrates 17.2 g
- Sugar 3.9 g
- Protein 4.4 g
- Cholesterol 0 mg

Ingredients:

- 2 sweet potatoes, wash, and cut into 1-inch pieces
- 1 lb Brussels sprouts, cut in half
- ¼ tsp chili powder
- 2 tbsp olive oil
- ¼ tsp garlic powder
- ½ tsp pepper
- 1 tsp salt

Directions:

1. Preheat the air fryer to 400 F.
2. Add sweet potatoes, Brussels sprouts, and remaining ingredients into the bowl and toss until well coated.
3. Transfer sweet potatoes and Brussels sprouts mixture into the air fryer basket and cook for 20 minutes. Stir halfway through.
4. Serve and enjoy.

Healthy Spinach Frittata

Preparation Time: 10 minutes

Cooking Time: 8 minutes

Serve: 1

Nutritional Value (Amount per Serving):

- Calories 190
- Fat 11.7 g
- Carbohydrates 4.3 g
- Sugar 3.3 g
- Protein 15.7 g
- Cholesterol 337 mg

Ingredients:

- 2 eggs, lightly beaten
- ¼ cup spinach, chopped
- ¼ cup tomatoes, chopped
- 2 tbsp almond milk

- ¼ tsp garlic powder
- 1 tbsp parmesan cheese, grated
- Pepper
- Salt

Directions:

1. In a bowl, whisk eggs. Add remaining ingredients and whisk until well combined.
2. Spray small air fryer pan with cooking spray.
3. Pour egg mixture into the prepared pan.
4. Place pan into the air fryer basket and cook at 330 F for 8 minutes.
5. Serve and enjoy.

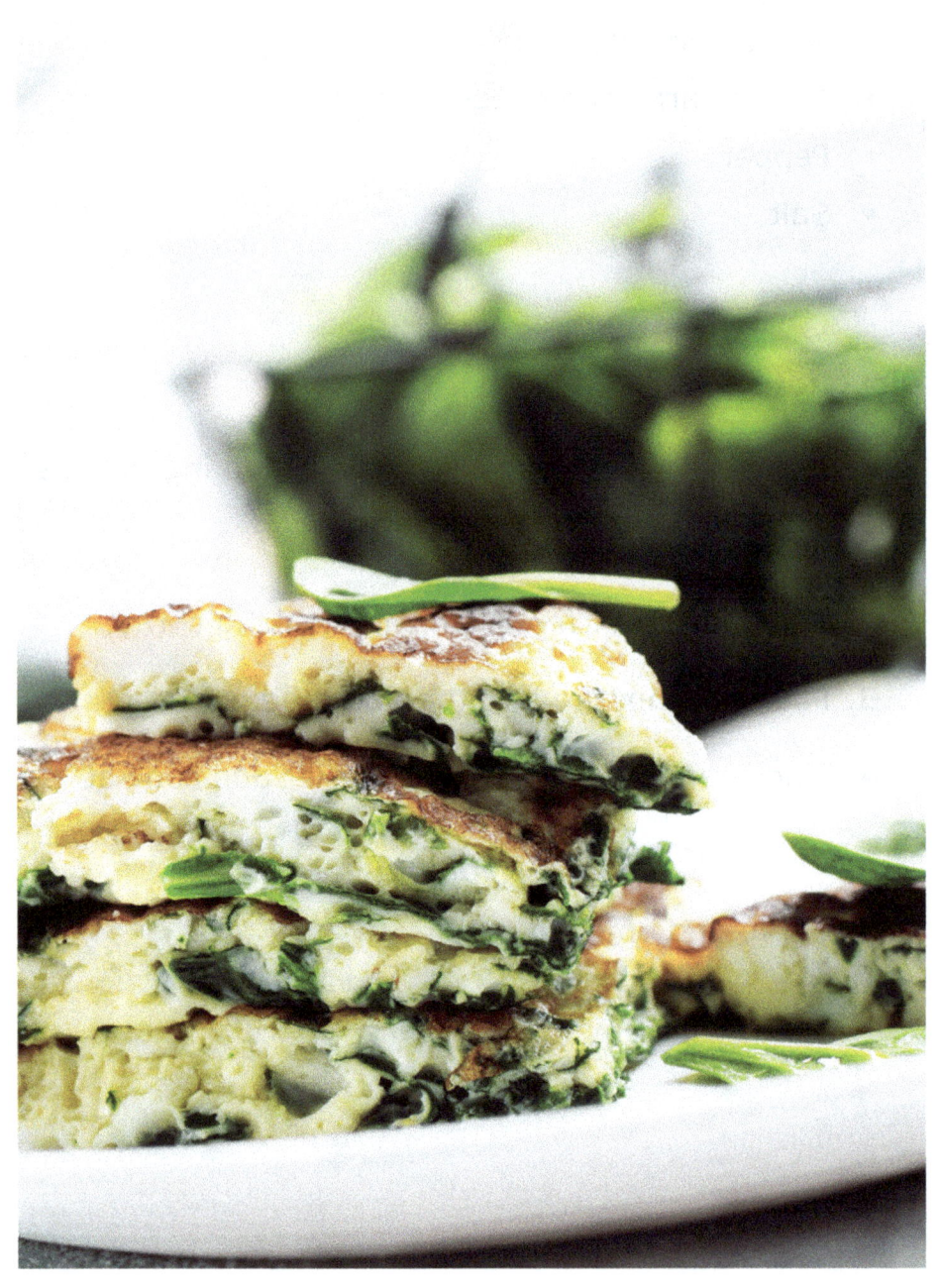

Breakfast Potatoes

Preparation Time: 10 minutes

Cooking Time: 20 minutes

Serve: 6

Nutritional Value (Amount per Serving):

- Calories 105
- Fat 2.5 g
- Carbohydrates 18.5 g
- Sugar 1.5 g
- Protein 2.1 g
- Cholesterol 0 mg

Ingredients:

- 1 ½ lbs potatoes, diced into ½-inch cubes
- ¼ tsp chili powder
- ¼ tsp pepper

- 1 tsp paprika
- 1 tsp garlic powder
- 1 tbsp olive oil
- Salt

Directions:

1. Add potatoes and remaining ingredients into the bowl and toss well.
2. Add potatoes into the air fryer basket and cook at 400 F for 20 minutes. Stir potatoes halfway through.
3. Serve and enjoy.

Spinach Pepper Egg Bites

Preparation Time: 10 minutes

Cooking Time: 20 minutes

Serve: 6

Nutritional Value (Amount per Serving):

- Calories 60
- Fat 4.2 g
- Carbohydrates 1.7 g
- Sugar 1.1 g
- Protein 4.1 g
- Cholesterol 109 mg

Ingredients:

- 4 eggs
- 1/2 cup spinach, chopped
- 1/2 cup roasted peppers, chopped

- 1/8 cup almond milk
- 2 tbsp green onion, chopped
- 1/4 tsp salt

Directions:

1. Preheat the air fryer to 325 F.
2. In a bowl, whisk eggs with milk and salt. Add spinach, green onion, and peppers and stir to combine.
3. Pour egg mixture into the silicone muffin molds.
4. Place muffin molds into the air fryer basket and cook for 12-15 minutes.
5. Serve and enjoy.

Egg Cheese Muffins

Preparation Time: 10 minutes

Cooking Time: 20 minutes

Serve: 6

Nutritional Value (Amount per Serving):

- Calories 165
- Fat 13.7 g
- Carbohydrates 1.4 g
- Sugar 0.4 g
- Protein 8.9 g
- Cholesterol 151 mg

Ingredients:

- 4 eggs
- 1 scoop whey protein powder
- 2 tbsp butter, melted

- 4 oz cream cheese
- Pepper
- Salt

Directions:

1. Preheat the air fryer to 325 F.
2. Add all ingredients into the bowl and whisk until combine.
3. Pour batter into the silicone muffin molds.
4. Place muffin molds into the air fryer basket and cook for 20 minutes.
5. Serve and enjoy.

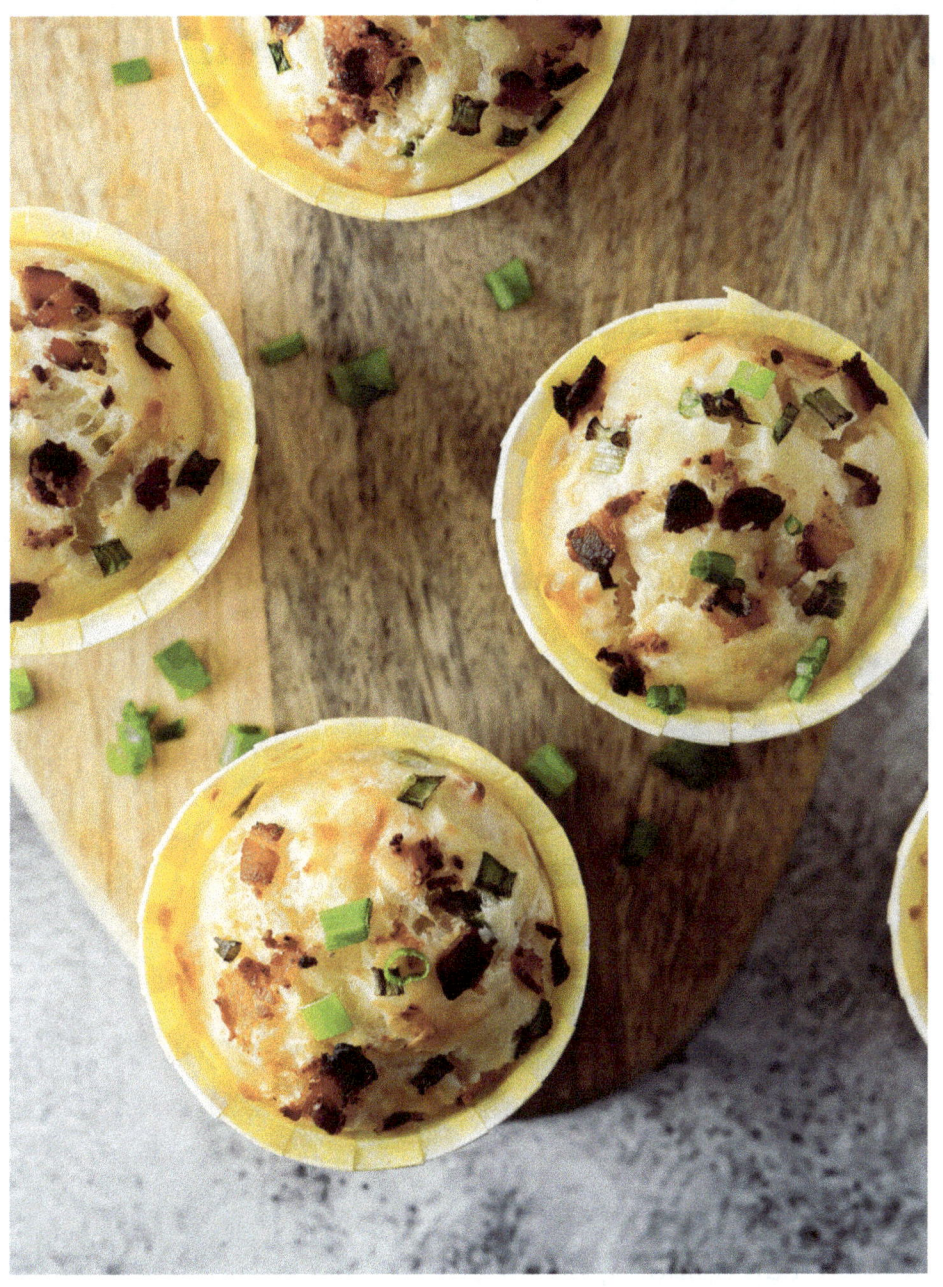

Mushroom Spinach Muffins

Preparation Time: 10 minutes

Cooking Time: 15 minutes

Serve: 6

Nutritional Value (Amount per Serving):

- Calories 75
- Fat 5 g
- Carbohydrates 0.9 g
- Sugar 0.5 g
- Protein 6.1 g
- Cholesterol 140 mg

Ingredients:

- 5 eggs
- 1 cup spinach, chopped
- 1/4 tsp onion powder

- 1/2 cup mushrooms, chopped
- 1/4 tsp garlic powder
- Pepper
- Salt

Directions:

1. Preheat the air fryer to 375 F.
2. In a bowl, whisk eggs with garlic powder, onion powder, pepper, and salt. Add spinach and mushrooms and stir well.
3. Pour egg mixture into the 6 silicone muffin molds.
4. Place muffin molds into the air fryer basket and cook for 10-12 minutes.
5. Serve and enjoy.

Egg Veggie Soufflé

Preparation Time: 10 minutes

Cooking Time: 20 minutes

Serve: 4

Ingredients:

- 4 eggs
- 1/2 cup mushrooms, chopped
- 1 tsp onion powder
- 1 tsp garlic powder
- 1/2 cup broccoli florets, chopped
- Pepper
- Salt

Nutritional Value (Amount per Serving):

- Calories 85
- Fat 5.1 g
- Carbohydrates 2.4 g

- Sugar 1.1 g
- Protein 7.1 g
- Cholesterol 186 mg

Directions:

1. Preheat the air fryer to 350 F.
2. Spray four ramekins with cooking spray and set aside.
3. In a bowl, whisk eggs with onion powder, garlic powder, pepper, and salt. Add mushrooms and broccoli and stir well.
4. Pour egg mixture into the prepared ramekins.
5. Place ramekins into the air fryer basket and cook for 20 minutes.
6. Serve and enjoy.

Italian Egg Muffins

Preparation Time: 10 minutes

Cooking Time: 20 minutes

Serve: 12

Nutritional Value (Amount per Serving):

- Calories 65
- Fat 4.4 g
- Carbohydrates 2.1 g
- Sugar 1.2 g
- Protein 4 g
- Cholesterol 87 mg

Ingredients:

- 6 eggs
- 3 cherry tomatoes, chopped
- 4 sun-dried tomatoes, chopped

- 1/2 cup feta cheese, crumbled
- 2 tsp olive oil
- Pepper
- Salt

Directions:

1. Preheat the air fryer to 350 F.
2. In a bowl, whisk eggs with pepper and salt. Add remaining ingredients and stir well.
3. Pour egg mixture into the 12 silicone muffin molds.
4. Place half muffin molds into the air fryer basket and cook for 12-15 minutes.
5. Serve and enjoy.

Marinated Ginger Garlic Salmon

Preparation Time: 10 minutes

Cooking Time: 10 minutes

Serve: 2

Nutritional Value (Amount per Serving):

- Calories 334
- Fat 18.2 g
- Carbohydrates 9 g
- Sugar 3.4 g
- Protein 35.7 g
- Cholesterol 78 mg

Ingredients:

- 2 salmon fillets, skinless & boneless

- 1 1/2 tbsp mirin
- 1 1/2 tbsp soy sauce
- 1 tbsp olive oil
- 2 tbsp green onion, minced
- 1 tbsp ginger, grated
- 1 tsp garlic, minced

Directions:

1. Add mirin, soy sauce, oil, green onion, ginger, and garlic into the zip-lock bag and mix well.
2. Add fish fillets into the bag, seal the bag, and place in the refrigerator for 30 minutes.
3. Preheat the air fryer to 360 F.
4. Spray air fryer basket with cooking spray.
5. Place marinated salmon fillets into the air fryer basket and cook for 10 minutes.
6. Serve and enjoy.

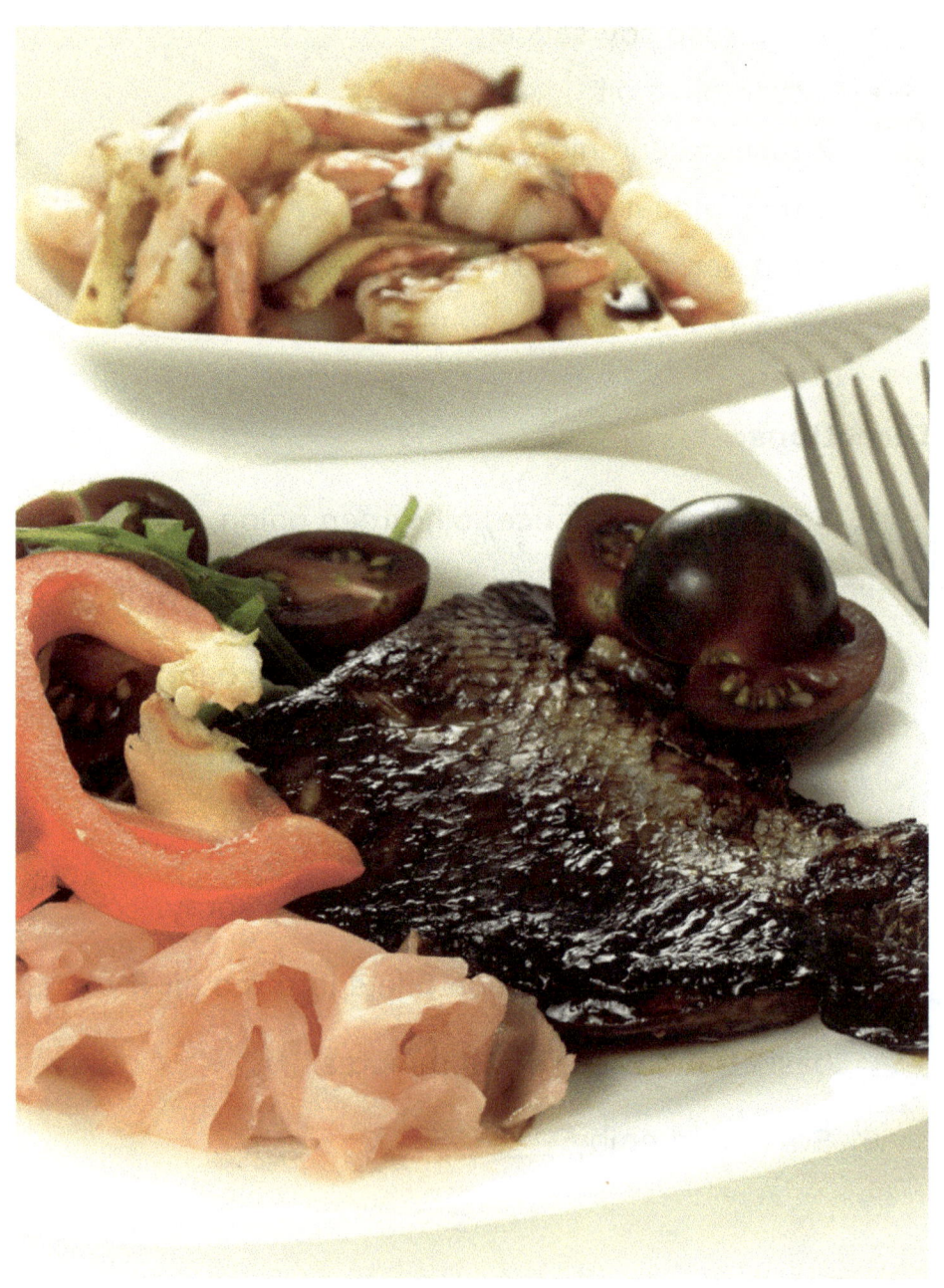

www.ingramcontent.com/pod-product-compliance
Lightning Source LLC
Chambersburg PA
CBHW070732030426
42336CB00013B/1945